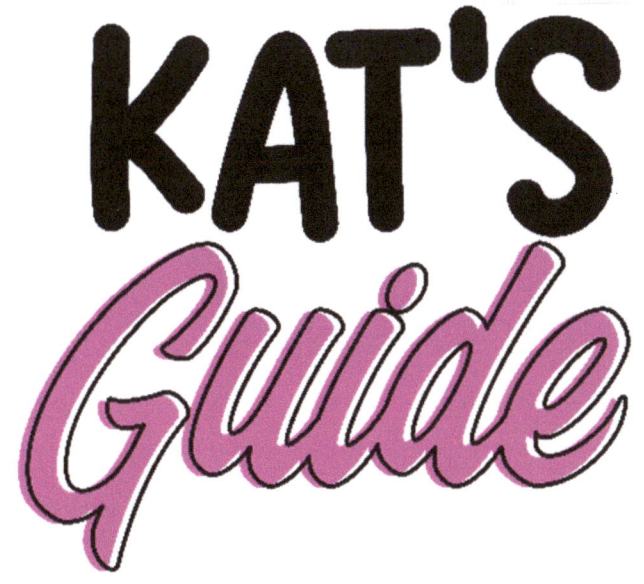

All About Hair

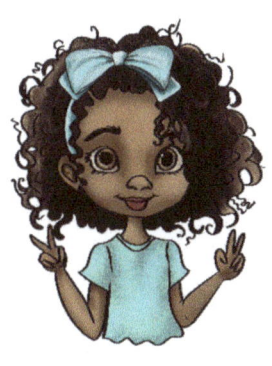

Bebe

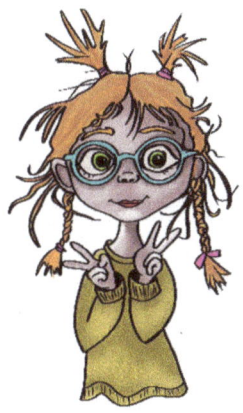

Lola

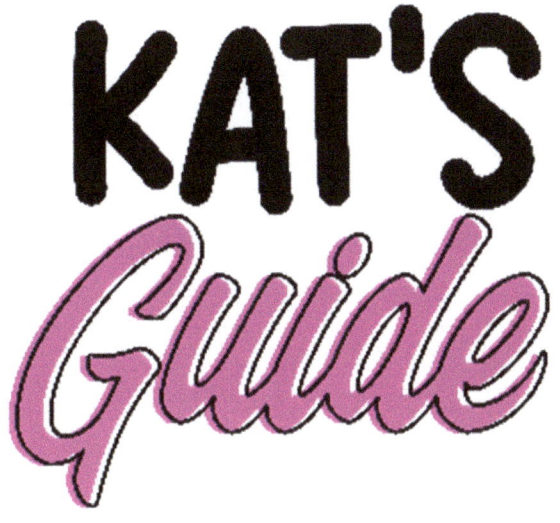

All About Hair

The Ultimate Guide to Healthy, Happy Hair for Girls

Copyright © 2025 by Kathryn Hinckley
Kat's Guide: All About Hair
All rights reserved.

No part of this publication may be reproduced, distributed, or transmitted in any form or by any means, including photocopying, recording, or other electronic or mechanical methods, without prior written permission of the publisher, except in the case of brief quotations embodied in critical reviews and certain other noncommercial uses permitted by copyright law.

Although the author and publisher have made every effort to ensure that the information in this book was correct at press time, the author and publisher do not assume and hereby disclaim any liability to any party for any loss, damage, or disruption caused by errors or omissions, whether such errors or omissions result from negligence, accident, or any other cause.

Adherence to all applicable laws and regulations, including international, federal, state and local governing professional licensing, business practices, advertising, and all other aspects of doing business in the US, Canada or any other jurisdiction is the sole responsibility of the reader and consumer.

Neither the author nor the publisher assumes any responsibility or liability whatsoever on behalf of the consumer or reader of this material. Any perceived slight of any individual or organization is purely unintentional. The resources in this book are provided for informational purposes only and should not be used to replace the specialized training and professional judgment of a health care or mental health care professional.

Paperback ISBN: 979-8-9851882-4-0

Moso Method Publishers
Sterling, MA

To order in bulk or inquire about interviews and media, contact the author at kathryn@mosomethod.com
Cover designer & Illustrations: Cutting Edge Studio

Dedication

For every girl who has ever stared in the mirror feeling frustrated with her hair...

For every messy bun that wasn't supposed to be messy...

For every tangle that felt like the end of the world...

For every braid that turned into a knot...

This book is for YOU!

Hair isn't hard - it just feels that way until you learn how to manage it.

And once you learn? GIRL, you've got it!

I'm Kathryn, and I've been helping people feel confident, creative, and in control of their hair for over 30 years. I'm a beauty industry professional who's done everything from wedding make-up to film industry hair and now, I'm going to share everything I've learned with YOU in Kat's Guide books.

This is your first step into the world of beauty, fun, and fearless hair days.

Because every future fashionista deserves to feel like a hair pro.

Now let's make magic happen - one braid, wash, or style at a time!

Kathryn

Table of Contents

You are: The Next Generation of Beauty 1

1. The Basics Hair Health 3

2. How to properly wash your hair 5

3. It's Clean, now what? 9

4. Your hair is AWESOME 13

5. Keeping Hair Healthy 23

6. Simple Styles 3 Strand Braid 27

7. Practice time 31

8. French Braid Glow-Up 35

9. Fun Hair Facts 41

10. Should I color my hair at home? NO!!! 43

11. Final Tips from Kat 49

Author Biography 53

You are:
The Next Generation of Beauty

Welcome to the wonderful world of hair! With over 30 years as a cosmetologist, my love for styling started when I was just a kid, playing with my doll's hair and dreaming up fun looks. Before I knew it, I was experimenting with friends and discovering the magic of transforming hair into something beautiful. Now, I'm here to share that spark with you!

This book is your introduction to the exciting world of hair, whether you're looking for a creative hobby or laying the foundation for a future career. From simple tips to fun techniques, you'll find everything you need to start exploring. So grab your hair tools, unleash your imagination, and let's dive into a world full of creativity, color, and style!

"Your passion - your fashion"

The Basics Hair Health

Taking care of your hair is like taking care of a superhero's cape - it's part of what makes you awesome! Healthy hair is strong, shiny, and feels great, but it needs a little love to stay that way. Think of your hair as a plant: it needs the right care and nutrients to grow and stay healthy. Your hair needs to be washed regularly to keep it clean, brushed gently to help it stay smooth, and nourished through eating healthy foods to give it the power to grow strong.

When you take care of your hair, you're also taking care of yourself! It's fun to try new styles, but overdoing things like heat or tight hairstyles can cause damage. Keep your hair healthy by using the right products and following the proper care and style tips from Kat's Guide. Treat your hair like a treasure - it's unique and special, just like you!

How to properly wash your hair

Washing your hair is like giving it a nice, bubbly bath, it keeps it clean, fresh, and happy! Here's how to do it the right way:

Wet your hair:

Start by soaking your hair with warm water (not too hot - it's not soup!). This helps loosen dirt and gets your hair ready for shampoo.

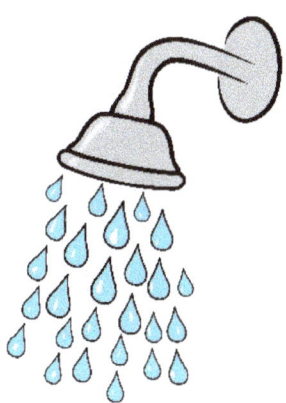

Shampoo your hair:

Squeeze a little shampoo into your hand (about the size of a coin) and rub your hands together to spread it out.

Then, gently massage it into your scalp with your fingertips - no scratching! This is where all the dirt and oils hang out, so give it a good scrub all over with the pads of your fingers. Be sure to lather over your ears and all around your hairline, too.

Pro Tip: If you'd like it to be more sudsy, try adding more water.

Rinse it out:

Rinse all the shampoo out with water until your hair feels squeaky clean. No bubbles left behind!

Leaving shampoo residue in your hair can make your scalp itchy (and nobody likes that!).

Condition your Hair:

Conditioner is like a special treat for your hair - it makes it soft and smooth! Put a small amount in your hands and apply it to the ends of your hair (not the roots- where your hair connects to your head). If you condition your scalp, it can get dirty faster. The ends need extra love because they can get dry. Let the conditioner hang out on your hair for a couple of minutes. I recommend washing and conditioning your hair and then washing your body while the conditioner works its magic. This is a great time to use a wide-toothed comb or wet brush to detangle your hair.

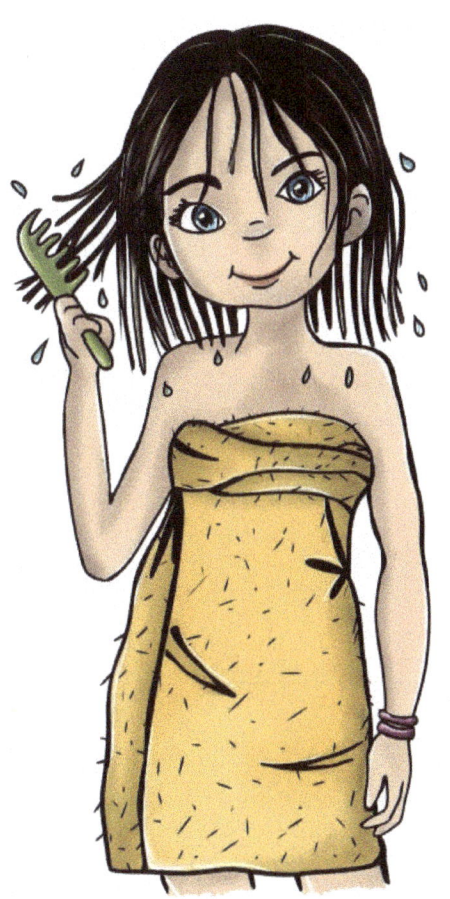

Rinse again:

After letting the conditioner sit for a minute or two, rinse it out completely with water.

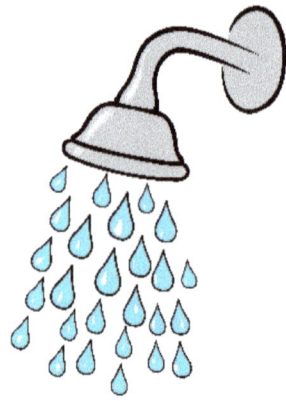

Conditioner residue can act like a magnet for dust and dirt, so rinse well.

It's Clean, now what?

After washing your hair, it's important to treat it gently and give it the care it needs to stay healthy and strong. Here's a fun, easy routine to follow:

Pat, don't rub! Use a soft microfiber towel or an old t-shirt to gently blot the water from your hair.

Avoid rubbing, as this can cause frizz and breakage.

Detangle with care. While your hair is still damp, use a wide-tooth comb, wet brush, or your fingers to gently remove tangles. Start at the ends and work your way up to avoid pulling or damaging your strands.

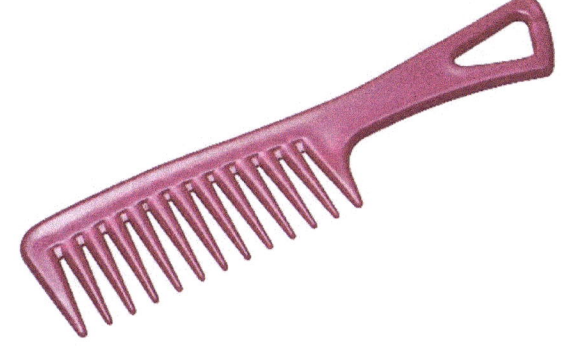

Pro Tip: When using a wet brush, hold it vertically (up and down) to more easily brush through tangles.

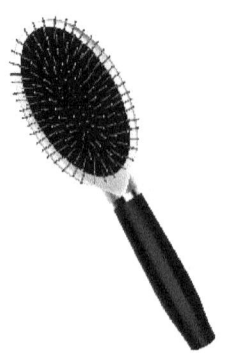

Add some love. Apply a leave-in conditioner or a lightweight serum to lock in moisture and keep your hair soft and shiny. This also makes styling easier!

Protect before the heat. If you plan to use a blow dryer or styling tools, always apply a heat protectant spray first to shield your hair from damage.

Air-dry when you can. Letting your hair air-dry is the healthiest option, but if you need to blow-dry, use the lowest heat setting and keep the dryer moving to prevent overheating.

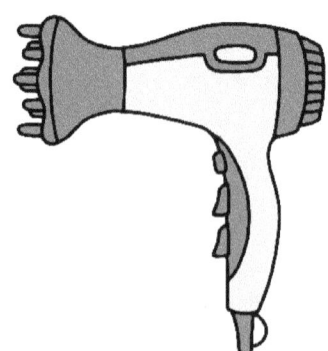

By following these steps, you'll keep your hair happy, healthy, and ready for any style you want to try!

Your hair is AWESOME

(Even if it doesn't look like your friends)

Let's make hair care fun and easy to understand! Think of your hair like a best friend - it has a personality all its own, and when you treat it right, it'll shine (literally). Here's a quick guide to different hair types, how to care for each type, and the various products that will make your hair the star of the show.

Hair Types & How to Care for Them

1. Fine Hair (The Skinny Friend)

Fine hair can feel thin and can get greasy fast, but it's also super soft. It sometimes needs a little boost to avoid looking flat.

Products: Volumizing shampoo, lightweight conditioner, root-lifting spray, and mousse.

<u>*How to Use:*</u>

Wash your hair 2-3 times a week with volumizing shampoo.

Apply conditioner only to the ends (not the roots - no one likes greasy roots!). Comb the conditioner through your hair, starting at your ends to avoid ripping through snarls. Use a wide-toothed comb or wet brush to prevent breakage. Make sure to rinse it out completely. Towel dry gently when finished.

Before blow-drying, spritz on root-lifting spray or mousse and dry upside down for extra volume (always use a heat protector and avoid any heavy products).

Try dry shampoo between washes if you're feeling dirty.

2. Coarse Hair (The Strong Rebel)

Coarse hair is thick and powerful but can be prone to dryness and frizz. It loves moisture!

Products: Moisturizing shampoo, moisturizing conditioner, deep conditioning masks, leave-in conditioner, styling cream, heat protector, and shine serum.

How to Use:

Wash 1-2 times a week with moisturizing shampoo. Apply moisturizing conditioner to the mid-section and ends of your hair. Use a wet brush or wide-toothed comb to distribute the product throughout your hair. Start from the ends to avoid pulling at tangles.

Use a deep conditioning mask every other week. Leave it on for 10 minutes while you check out my posts on Tik-Tok @kathinckley. Gently rinse, towel dry to remove most of the moisture. If you are using a leave-in conditioner, this is the time to apply it.

Apply a nickel-sized amount of styling cream to your ends first, moving up your hair to about 1 inch away from your scalp. Use a turban or wrap an old t-shirt around your head to remove most of the moisture. Diffuse your hair while scrunching (squeezing your hair and gently lifting toward your scalp).

Rub a small drop (size of a pea) of a shine serum or argan oil between your palms and smooth it onto dry hair for shine and softness.

Try using a satin pillowcase to help it stay smoother longer.

3. Dry Hair (The Thirsty Diva)

Dry hair craves hydration like you crave snacks after school.

Products: Hydrating shampoo, deep conditioning mask, leave-in conditioner, shine serum, and hydrating spray.

How to Use:

Wash your hair with hydrating shampoo twice a week.

Use a deep conditioning mask every other week - leave on for 10 minutes. I recommend washing and conditioning your hair and then washing your body while the conditioner works its magic. This is a great time to use a wide-toothed comb or wet brush to detangle your hair.

Spray on leave-in conditioner after washing, focus on the ends!

Air dry your hair as often as possible. If you must blow dry, use moderate heat and be sure to always use a heat protector.

Try keeping a hydrating spray in your bag for quick spritzes during the day.

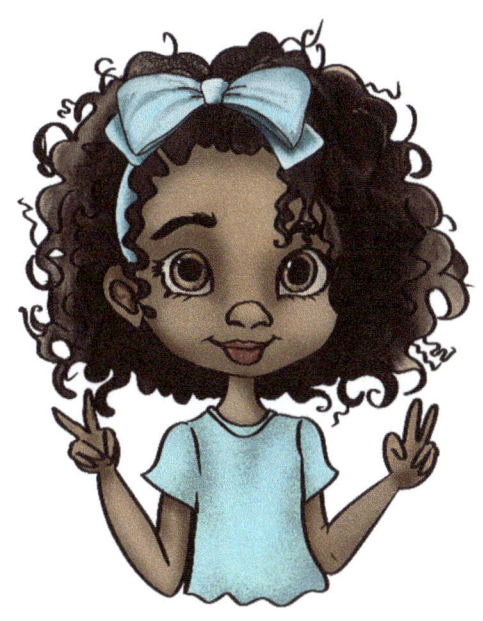

4. Damaged Hair (The Drama Queen)

If you've been straightening, curling, or dyeing like crazy, your hair might be feeling stressed out. Yes! Your hair can feel stressed out too, but you can calm it down with these tips.

Products: Repairing shampoo, protein treatments, leave-in conditioner, heat protectant, and shine serum.

<u>How to Use:</u>

Wash with repairing shampoo twice a week to strengthen weak strands. Spray on leave-in conditioner, focusing on the ends and mid-section of your hair.

Every two weeks, use a protein treatment, follow the instructions on the bottle - **do not overuse**, or you can hurt your hair more.

Before using *any* heat tools (yes, even your blow dryer), apply heat protectant spray.

Try getting a haircut every 6 weeks to get rid of dead and damaged ends more frequently.

5. Frizzy Hair (The Wild Child)

Frizzy hair has a mind of its own, especially when it's humid, but don't worry! You can tame it.

Products: Moisturizing shampoo, deep conditioner, leave-in conditioner, anti-frizz serum, curl cream (if curly), smoothing serum, hair oils.

<u>*How to Use:*</u>

Wash with moisturizing shampoo and deep conditioner 2-3 times per week. Spritz in leave-in conditioner if extra moisturizing is needed.

Apply anti-frizz serum to damp hair before styling.

If you have curls or waves, apply a nickel-sized amount of curl cream while your hair is still wet, starting at the ends of your hair. Let your hair dry naturally, or use a diffuser attachment on your hair dryer to help define your curls (make sure to use a heat protector if blow drying).

Curly hair loves to be "scrunched"! To help define your curls, scrunch your hair while it's air drying or being blow-dried by squeezing sections of your hair while lifting up gently. You can even hang your head upside down and scrunch your hair up to your scalp.

Finish with shine serum or hair oil for sleekness that lasts all day.

Pro Tip: Try to avoid touching curly hair once it's dry to keep it looking its best throughout the day.

6. Flat or Limp Hair (The Chill One)

Flat hair needs some energy! Think of it as giving your hair a pep talk.

Products: Protein shampoo or Volumizing shampoo, protein conditioner, volumizing mousse or sea salt spray, heat protector.

How to Use:

Shampoo and condition 3-4 times a week.

Work volumizing mousse into damp roots before blow-drying, always use heat protector.

Try spritzing sea salt spray onto dry or damp hair and scrunch with your hands for fun, beachy vibes.

Bonus Tips for All Hair Types:

Don't over-wash! Washing too often can strip natural oils that keep your scalp happy.

Always use lukewarm water (not hot) to avoid drying out your strands.

Apply styling products to wet hair and comb through for even distribution.

Trim those ends every 6-8 weeks to keep split ends away!

Protect from heat! Your flat iron isn't evil if you use a heat protectant first.

***If your hair gets extra flat in damp weather**, your hair needs more protein.

***If your hair gets frizzy in damp weather**, your hair needs more moisture.

Keeping Hair Healthy

Your hair needs love even while you're catching your Z's! Taking care of your hair while you sleep helps keep it healthy, smooth, and tangle-free.

Here's how to make **bedtime hair care fun:**

Braids for bedtime: If you have long hair, try a loose braid before bed - it's like giving your hair a cozy hug! Braids (which you'll be learning soon) keep your hair from tangling and breaking while you sleep. Plus, you'll wake up with fun waves in the morning!

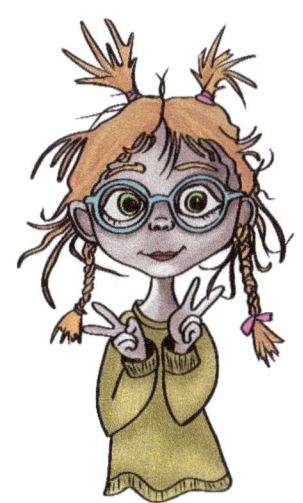

Sleep bonnet magic: A sleep bonnet is like a superhero cape for your hair! Made of soft satin or silk, it protects your strands from rubbing against your pillow and keeps your hair smooth and shiny overnight. Bonus: it feels fancy!

Pillow power: If bonnets aren't your style, switch to a satin or silk pillowcase. It's gentle on your hair and helps prevent frizz and breakage (I promise your head won't slide off).

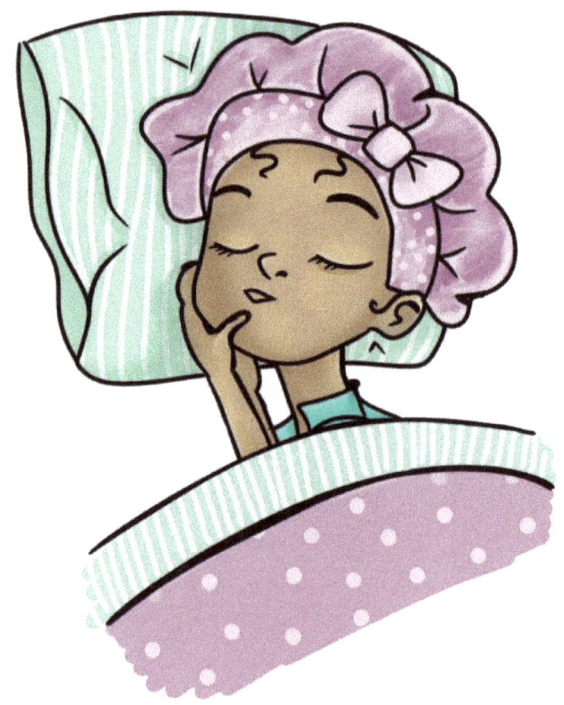

And don't forget about **sun protection!** Just like your skin, your hair needs protection from the sun's rays. If you're spending time outside, wear a hat or use a leave-in conditioner with UV protection to keep your hair safe from damage.

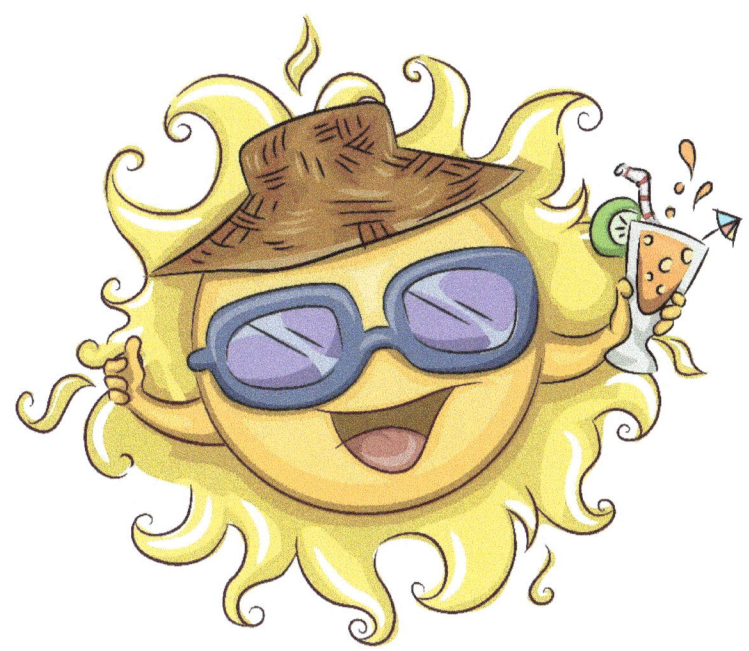

Taking care of your hair while sleeping and playing in the sun keeps it healthy and happy, because even superheroes (and their capes) need rest and protection!

Simple Styles 3 Strand Braid

(the blueprint for braid magic)

Now we get to the fun part - styling your hair! Let's start with a classic and super simple style: the 3-strand braid. It's easy to learn, looks great, and is perfect for keeping your hair neat and stylish. The 3-strand braid is the OG of all braids. Learn this, and your braid art has no limits!

Prep your hair: Brush your hair to make sure it's smooth and tangle-free. You can braid all of your hair or just a small section - your choice!

Divide into three sections: Separate the hair you want to braid into three equal pieces. Hold two sections in one hand and the third section in your other hand. In your mind name them, left - middle - right.

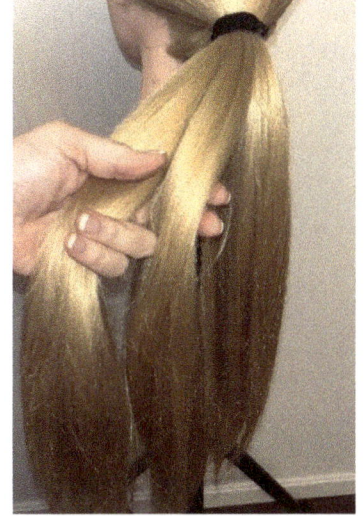

Start braiding: Take the section on the right and cross it over the middle section - it becomes the new middle piece! Then take the section on the left and cross it over the new middle piece (braiding is simply taking the outside pieces and making them the middle piece, one side at a time).

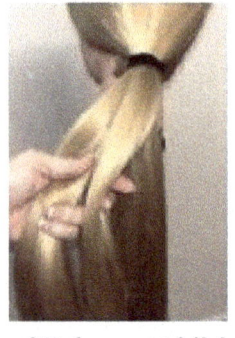 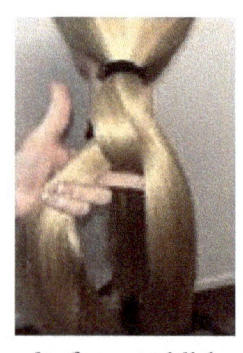 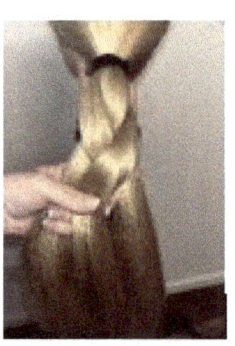

(Right to middle)   *(Left to middle)*   *(Right to middle)*

Repeat: Keep crossing the right section over the middle, then the left section over the middle, all the way down until you reach the end of your hair.

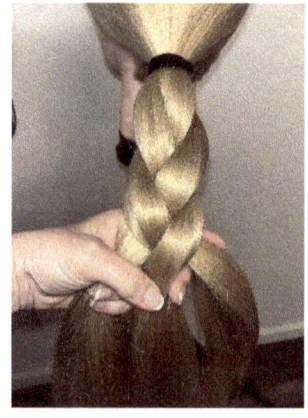

Secure it: Once you've braided down till you run out of hair, tie it off with a hair elastic to keep it in place.

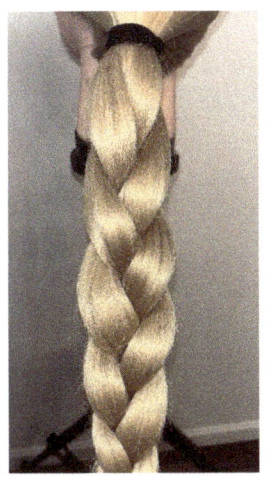

Voilà! You've created a beautiful 3-strand braid! Practice makes perfect, so try it a few times until you get the hang of it. Once you master this braid, you'll be ready to explore even more fun styles!

As described, this is considered a V-style braid, the type of braid you see in a typical French-style braid (which we will get to soon).

Practice time

A great way to practice braiding is to start with something simple and manageable. Here are some fun and effective methods to help you master the technique:

Practice on a doll or mannequin head: If you have a doll or a practice mannequin, use it to get comfortable with the motions of braiding. Their hair stays still, making it easier to focus on your technique.

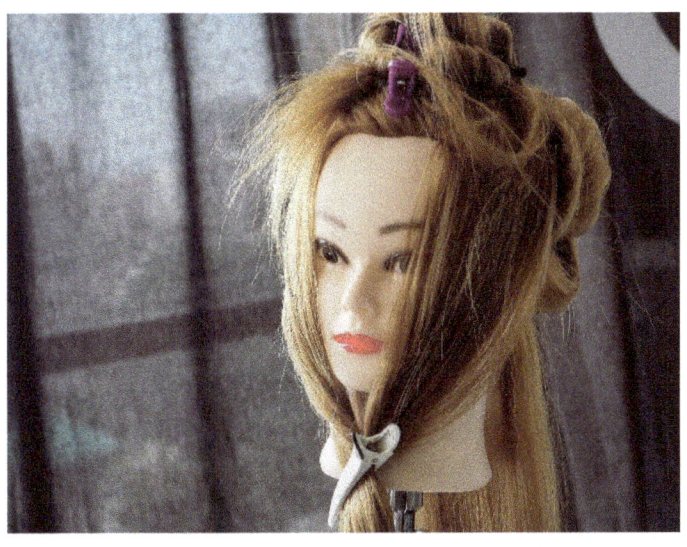

A little freaky but it gets the job done!

Use yarn or string: Learning on yarn or string is an excellent way to understand the basic crisscross motion without worrying about tangles. Tie three strands of string to a stable surface and practice crossing them over each other like you would with hair. To get an even better understanding, use three different colors of yarn to easily follow the pattern.

Try braiding a friend's hair: Ask a friend or family member if you can braid their hair. It's easier to learn on someone else's hair because you can see what you're doing clearly.

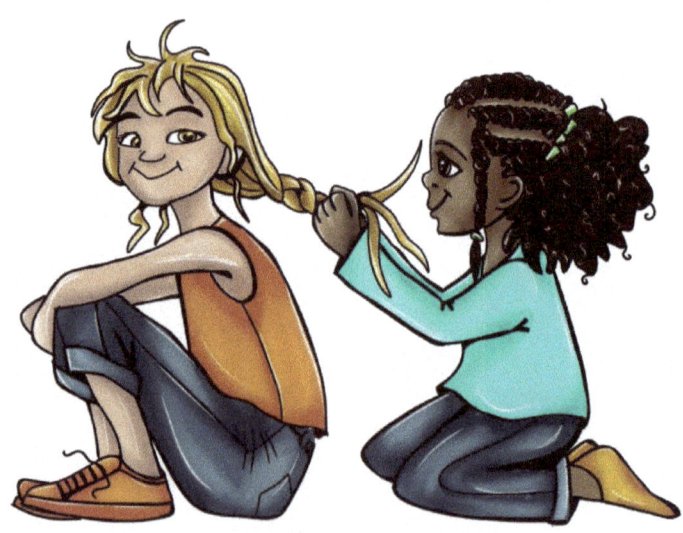

Work on your hair: Once you feel confident, practice braiding your hair in front of a mirror. Start with small sections until you get the hang of holding and crossing the strands properly.

Dedicate time for repetition: Set aside time each day to practice braiding. The more you repeat the motions, the faster your hands will learn the rhythm and pattern.

With consistent practice, you'll be creating neat and stylish braids in no time!

French Braid Glow-Up

Learning how to turn a simple 3-strand braid into a French braid is like leveling up your hair game - it's easier than it looks and super fun once you get the hang of it!

Let's break it down step-by-step so you can become a braiding pro in no time.

Simple strands today, total braid queen tomorrow!

Step 1: Start with the Basics

First, brush your hair to make sure there are no tangles (nobody likes a knotty surprise mid-braid). Then, grab a section of hair from the top of your head, near your forehead. This is your "starter section," and you'll divide it into three equal pieces, just like you would for a regular 3-strand braid.

Step 2: Begin the Braid

Start braiding like normal:

Cross the right strand over the middle strand.

Then cross the left strand over the new middle strand.

Boom - you've got the beginning of a regular braid. Easy, right?

Step 3: Add Some Hair Magic

Here's where things get fancy! Each time you cross a strand over the middle, grab a small piece of loose hair from the side of your head and add it to that strand before crossing it over.

When you cross the right strand over, grab some loose hair from the right side and add it to that strand.

When you cross the left strand over, grab some loose hair from the left side and add it to that strand.

It's like feeding your braid little snacks as you go!

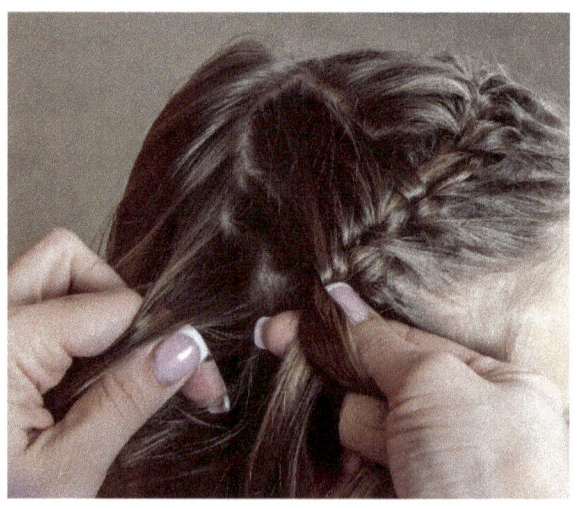

Step 4: Keep it going:

Repeat Step 3 down your head, adding more hair each time you cross a strand. Once you run out of loose hair (usually around your neck), just finish with a regular 3-strand braid and tie it off with an elastic.

The alternative is crossing the strands UNDERNEATH, as opposed to OVER the middle piece. This is considered an A-style braid, the type of braid you see in a typical Dutch-style braid

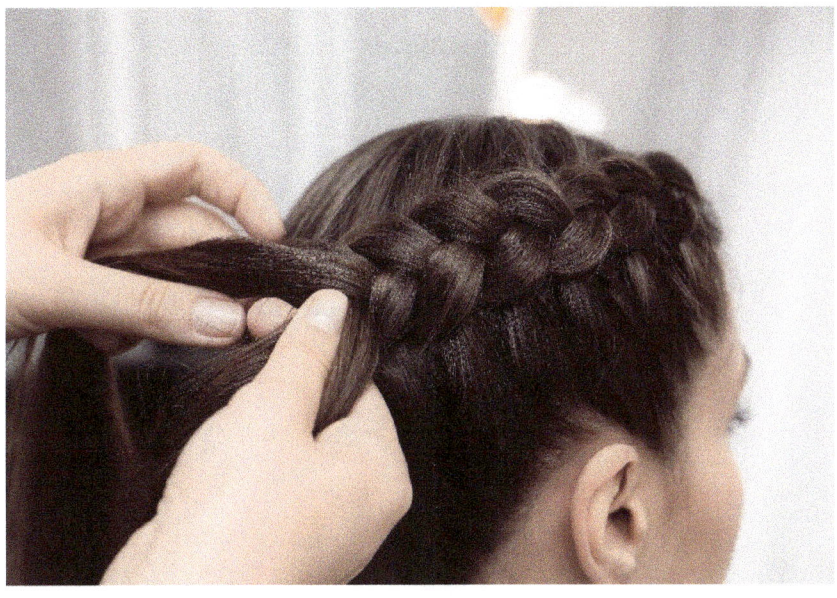

Pro Tips for Braiding Like a Boss

Practice Makes Perfect: Don't worry if it feels tricky at first - it's like learning to ride a bike for your fingers!

Use a Mirror: If you're braiding your hair, set up two mirrors so you can see what's happening in the back.

Keep It Tight: Pull each section snug as you go to keep your braid neat and secure.

Add Some Flair: Once you've mastered the French braid, try fun variations like double French braids or adding ribbons for extra style points!

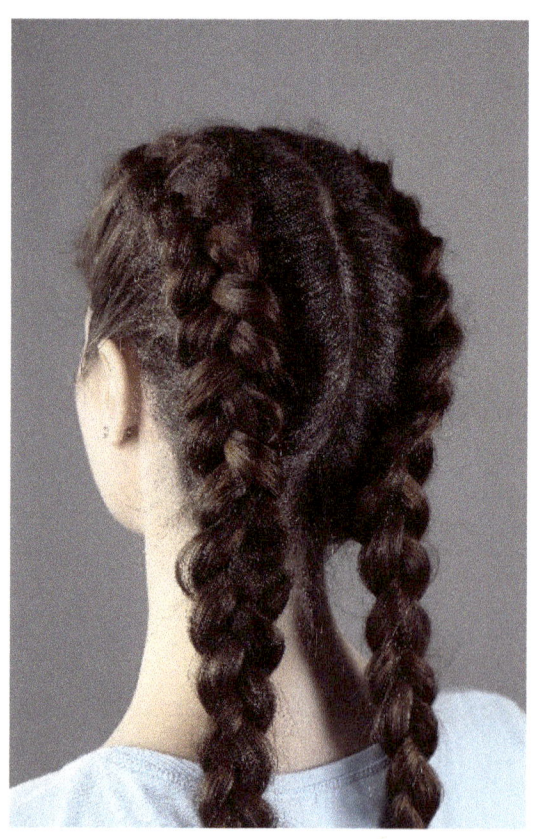

French braids are like magic - they take practice, but once you get them down, they look so cool and can be worn anywhere. So grab a brush, channel your inner stylist, and get braiding! You've got this!

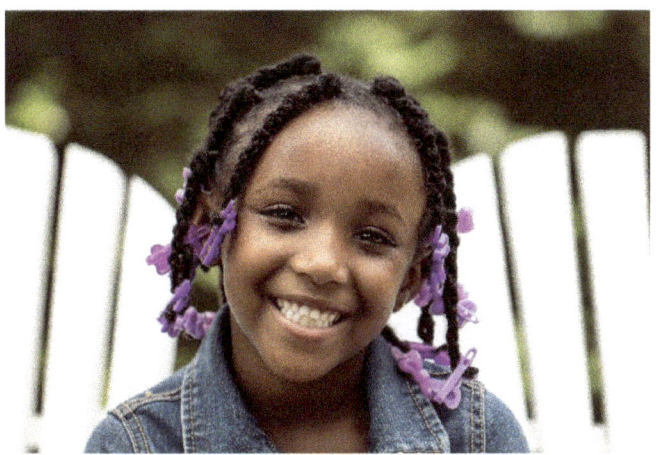

Fun Hair Facts

- The average person loses 50-150 strands a day.
- Black hair is the most common hair color in the world. Red hair is the rarest.
- Cutting hair does not affect hair growth.
- Hair grows an average of 1/2" per month.
- Hair grows faster in the summer.
- Evidence of everything that has been in your bloodstream, such as medicine, drugs, minerals, and vitamins, is traceable in your hair.
- The only thing that cannot be identified by hair is gender.
- Healthy hair can be stretched up to 30% of its length when wet (notice how long it gets in the pool?)
- If you counted all the growth of all the hairs on an average person's head, in one year, it would equate to over 10 miles of hair growth!
- Hair is the fastest-growing tissue in the body.

- A strand of hair is stronger than a copper wire of the same diameter.
- The average lifespan of an eyelash is 150 days.

Should I color my hair at home? NO!!!

Why You Shouldn't Play Mad Scientist with Your Hair at Home

You're staring at that box of dye or bleach, thinking, "How hard can it be?"

Well, let me stop you right there, because your hair is NOT a Pinterest craft project. Coloring or bleaching your hair at home might sound like a fun idea, but it's basically like trying to bake a cake without a recipe - you might get lucky, but chances are, it'll be a hot mess.

Here's why:

1. Bleach Is Like Fire On Your Hair

Bleach isn't some magical potion that turns you into a blonde bombshell—it's a super strong chemical that can totally roast your hair if you don't know what you're doing. Leave it on too long? Say hello to crispy, fried strands that snap off like dry spaghetti. Use too much? You might end up with patchy spots that look like a leopard print gone wrong. And don't even get me started on the potential scalp burns (ouch!).

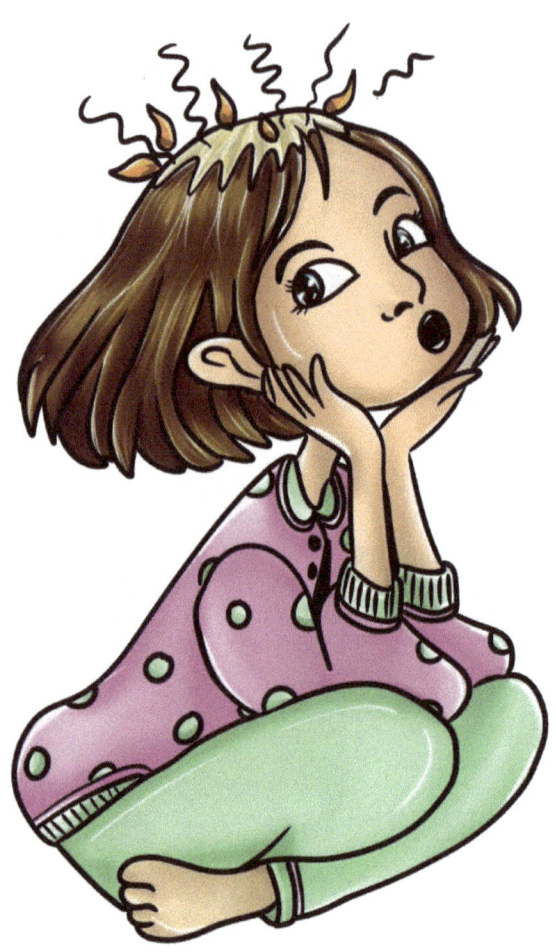

2. Box Dye Is the Ultimate Catfish

You know how sometimes online shopping looks amazing in the pictures but shows up looking NOTHING like what you ordered? That's box dye in a nutshell. The color on the box is lying to your face - it doesn't account for your hair's natural shade, texture, or condition. You wanted caramel brown? Surprise! You're now rocking streaky orange or muddy green. Cute… not.

3. DIY Hair Drama = $$$

Here's the real kicker: fixing a DIY color disaster costs way more than just going to a pro in the first place. Imagine spending hours trying to fix your mistake with more products (that probably won't work) and then having to beg a stylist to save your hair anyway. Spoiler alert: they'll charge extra because fixing fried or patchy hair is no easy task.

4. Your Hair Deserves Better!

Your hair is your crown - it deserves love and care, not chemical chaos in your bathroom sink. Professionals know exactly how to mix colors and apply bleach safely without turning your hair into straw or giving you zebra stripes.

So What Can You Do Instead?

Don't worry - I'm not here to crush your dream of switching up your look! There are so many fun ways to experiment without risking a hair disaster:

🎨 **Temporary Colors Are Your BFF:** Try hair chalks, sprays, or wash-out dyes for bold colors that vanish after a few shampoos - perfect for testing out pinks, blues, or purples without commitment!

🌈 **Clip-In Extensions:** Want highlights or funky colors? Clip-ins give you instant glam without touching your real hair. Plus, you can take them out whenever you want!

✨ **Wigs Are Everything:** Channel your inner superstar with wigs in every color of the rainbow - no damage, no stress, just instant fabulousness.

💖 **Accessorize Like a Pro:** Add some sparkle with glitter gel, colorful headbands, or funky barrettes. Sometimes all you need is a little bling!

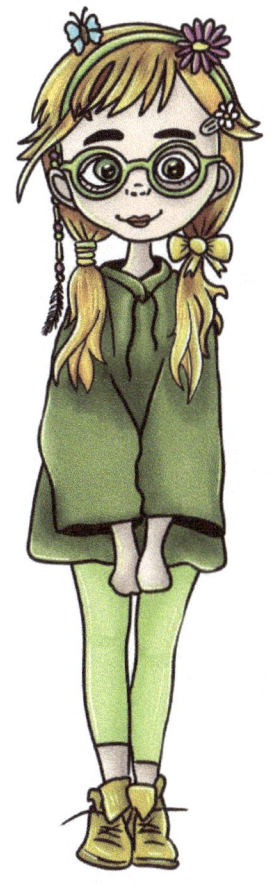

Pro Tip: Do NOT rip your elastics or scrunchies out of your hair. When you do that, you rip at your strands causing breakage that can't be fixed without a cut. Be gentle when removing any accessories.

The Bottom Line

DIY hair coloring sounds fun until it isn't - and trust me, fried hair isn't cute on anyone. If you're ready for a big change, call up a pro who knows how to safely make your dream look happen.

Until then, stick with temporary options and fun accessories - you'll still slay without risking your gorgeous locks.

So step away from the bleach bottle and grab some glitter instead - you're too fabulous for fried hair! ✨🎉

Final Tips from Kat

1. Be Gentle With Your Hair

Treat your hair like your favorite sweater - soft, loved, and never yanked! Use wide-tooth combs, pat instead of rub, and skip the tug-of-war.

2. Love Your Texture

Straight, curly, coily, wavy - every hair type is fabulous. Your hair's texture is part of your magic, so rock it with pride!

3. Hydration = Hair Happiness

Drink water. Use conditioner. Repeat. Moisture is your mane's BFF.

4. Don't Fear the Trim

Snipping off split ends doesn't mean losing length - it means making room for healthy growth! ✂️

5. Accessories Make Everything Better

Hair clips, headbands, scrunchies, beads, glitter gel... yes please! Go wild, go bold, go YOU! 🎀

6. Nighttime = Haircare Time

Satin pillowcases, loose braids, and sleep bonnets are like pajamas for your hair. Rest and protect those strands while you dream big!

7. No One's Born a Pro

Practice your braids. Try new styles. Mess up, laugh, and try again. Even stylists (like me!) started with a few "oops" moments - and even still have them.

8. Confidence Is the Best Product You Can Wear

No matter your style, your vibe, or your hair goals, confidence will always be your best look 💖

Keep Learning. Keep Playing. Keep Shining.

Your hair is a canvas. You are the artist.

THE END

Letter to the Reader

Congratulations, you made it to the end of Kat's Guide: All About Hair!

You are officially a hair care rockstar!

From learning how to detangle like a pro to trying out simple braids, to stylist-level french-braids, you've just leveled up in your hair game. Whether your hair is curly, coily, wavy, or straight, it's 100% YOU, and that makes it 100% AWESOME.

But guess what? This is just the beginning of your hair adventure! There's a whole world of styles to try, tips to learn, and fabulous hair days ahead. So keep experimenting, keep asking questions, and most of all—keep having fun with it!

Remember, your hair isn't just something on your head—it's part of your story. It's how you express yourself, show off your creativity, and share a little sparkle with the world. So wear it with pride, care for it with love, and never stop being your amazing, unstoppable self.

Until next time, stay curious, stay confident, and never be afraid to rock your unique, beautiful vibe.

Big hugs and even bigger hair,

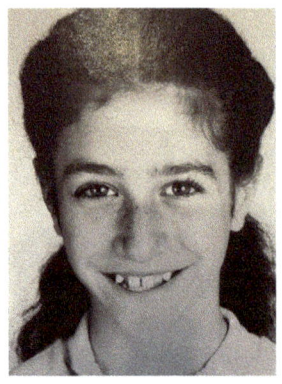 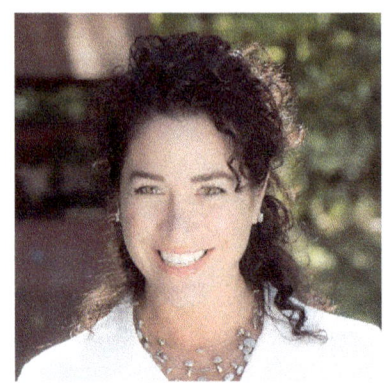

❤️ The Stylist Kat

Wanna stay in touch? I'd love to hear from you!

Tag your styles, tips, and selfies using #KatsGuide and find me @kat.moso.method.

Let's celebrate your fabulous hair journey together!

Oh—and keep an eye out for more Kat's Guide books.

You can find me at www.katsguide.com

Author Biography

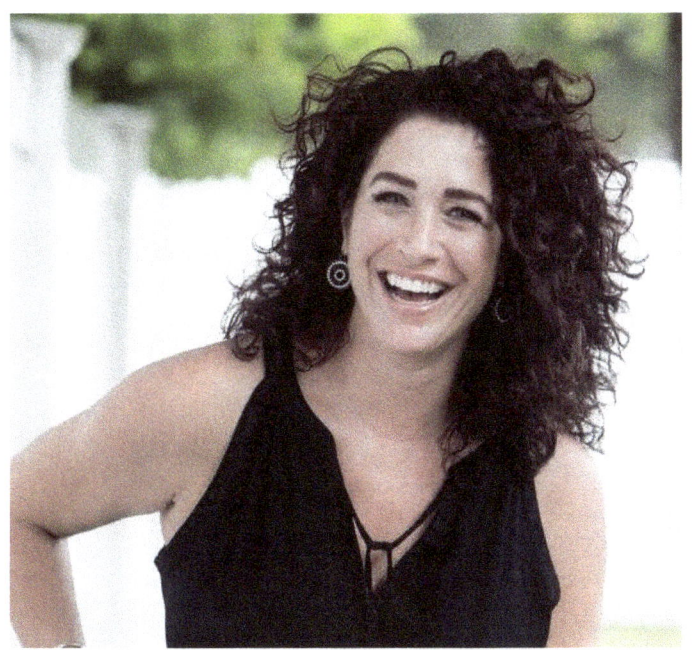

Kathryn Hinckley is a beauty industry powerhouse with a heart of gold - and a whole lot of hairspray. With over 30 years of experience as a stylist, educator, and global business leader, she's helped thousands of people feel confident from the inside out. From her early days behind the chair to managing international beauty brands, Kathryn has always believed in the power of great hair and an even greater mindset.

As the creator of *The Moso Method*, a breakthrough system for personal and professional growth, Kathryn brings her signature blend of wisdom, wit, and motivation to every workshop, coaching session, and bestselling book. Her mission? To help people uncover their unique sparkle and lead with purpose, positivity, and a little bit of flair.

Kathryn is also a proud mom in a blended family and loves nothing more than cheering on her crew, whether it's at home or from across the country. Her love for family, personal development, and meaningful connection shines through in everything she does.

Her debut kids' book, *Kat's Guide: All About Hair*, is a fun, feel-good guide to healthy hair and self-love. Kathryn believes great hair days are magic - but a strong sense of self? That's where the real glow starts.

She currently lives in the U.S. and continues to travel, teach, and light up rooms (and salons!) with her passion for people, beauty, and the magic of believing in yourself.

www.ingramcontent.com/pod-product-compliance
Lightning Source LLC
Chambersburg PA
CBHW052131030426
42337CB00028B/5116